99 Things to Know When You Have Breast Cancer

by

Melanie Payne

99 Things to Know When
You Have Breast Cancer

For Marla

Introduction

When you're diagnosed with breast cancer the doctors will talk about "staging." This means the severity of your cancer. Stage 0 isn't even cancer at all, some will say. Ask anyone who has had Stage 0 and they will beg to differ. Stage IV means it's spread throughout your body. But it doesn't mean your life is over. Many people live for years, even more than a decade, with this diagnosis.

I think people experience cancer in four different types of stages. The stage when you first get diagnosed. The stage when you're going through treatment. The stage when you're recovering from it. And the stage when you're living as a survivor of breast cancer.

I've compiled these tips for women. I know some of the people going through breast cancer are men, but let's face it, the overwhelming numbers of people who get breast cancer are women. So it's not that men can't learn something from these tips because they can. But this is a book from one woman to another.

And it's short. Because I realize if you are reading this book, you aren't interested in the "War and Peace" of breast cancer. You want to know what's ahead. You want some advice. You need suggestions. I also wanted this to be short enough that you could read the whole thing in one sitting. Because even though you are in Stage 1 of this trip (some call it a journey but that just sounds too pleasant) you need to know where it's going to lead you. And some of the 99 things, can be used at each stage, even if I didn't put them in until the end.

This is by no means everything you need to know about breast cancer. And some of these tips might not even apply to you. Some you might think are crazy or just plain wrong. If so, ignore them. But I think most of you, my sisters who have been diagnosed as having breast cancer, can find use for them.

I went through these stages myself. I felt so alone even though I knew I wasn't. I felt like a loser. A woman who drew the short straw. I was also confused and afraid. And that was the worst.

I wanted someone to tell me what I needed to do. What the future would hold for me. And most of all, I wanted someone to tell me I was going to be

OK. And I am. I'm not finished with breast cancer, but it no longer occupies my every waking moment. I'm not obsessed with it anymore. I'm not spending hours on the Internet. I stopped crying. I'm happy again.

I made it through breast cancer, you will too.

Stage I

Diagnosis

Get Ready

1

Most of the women diagnosed with breast cancer don't die of breast cancer.

2

Don't rush into anything. Very few decisions about what to do after you have been diagnosed with breast cancer have to be made right away. Ask your doctor if your surgery is an emergency or just urgent. If it's the latter, then wait and take some time to make decisions.

3

Read everything you can get your hands on. But don't believe everything you read.

4

If you can find a breast cancer navigator in your town, make an appointment to go see her. She is a specialist in breast cancer and can help you make decisions and give you the information on doctors, resources, research and options. She's invaluable.

5

Talk to other women who have had breast cancer. Their experience is not the same as yours although there will be similarities. Their outcome may be better. Or it may be worse. You'll learn from them.

6

There are way worse things you could be diagnosed with. Inoperable brain tumor, Lou Gherig's disease, AIDS, Alzheimer's – I'd rather have breast cancer than any of those.

7

Feel comfortable with your doctor. If you don't – find another. If there's an ounce of doubt in your mind, move on. Remember you pay them, they don't pay you.

8

Even if you love your doctor get a second opinion. If your doctor is a good one, she won't mind. If she does object, get another doctor.

9

Everyone will start asking if there is anything they can do. You want to say, "Give me back my life." They can't do that. Ask for something. Anything. It makes people feel useful and it gets them to leave you alone.

10

Get your financial house in order. Resist the urge to spend frivolously. You are going to need the money.

11

Even though you might need to be more frugal, don't deny yourself things that are going to make you feel better.

12

If your breast cancer is in the right breast, start practicing doing things with your left hand. If it's in your left, start using your right. After surgery being a little bit ambidextrous is a benefit.

13

Buy a couple new shirts that button down the front.

14

See a nurse who knows something about lymphedema and find out what you can do to prevent it.

15

You will hear, "It's your decision" over and over. Resist the temptation to say, "If I had any damn choice in the matter, I wouldn't have breast cancer."

16

Advice is plentiful but not much of it is useful.

17

No one's situation is exactly like yours.

18

Everyone you meet knows someone who had breast cancer. Just because their mother, friend or sister died, it doesn't mean you will.

19
Don't ask, "Why me?" Ask, "Why not me?"

20
There's still something to laugh about every day.

21
There are almost always at least two choices. Always ask what the other option is. You don't have to exercise it, but you should know it.

22
Don't forget that your spouse, partner, and other significant people in your life might be afraid too.

23
Don't have a mastectomy if the only thing you think it will do is buy you peace of mind. It won't.

24
Bring a nice wool shawl with you to all appointments. You'll be surprised how cold it can be sitting in an office wearing only a gown.

25
Don't listen to anyone who tells you not to go on the Internet for information or support.

26
Remember, the Internet is often full of trash when it comes to breast cancer, ignore a lot of it.

27

Call your friends and tell them you want to talk about your cancer.

28

Don't put off too long telling good friends you have breast cancer. It's an easier conversation to have than it is explaining to them a year later that you didn't want them to know or having them hear about it from someone else.

29

If you like to read, you'll have plenty of time to do it. Invest in an electronic book reader. It's easy to carry around, you can choose what you want to read and don't have to rely on whatever is in the waiting rooms.

30

You will feel depressed. If you don't feel a little down about being diagnosed with breast cancer, something really is wrong.

Stage II

Treatment

Get it taken care of.

31
A dog is a great comfort when you don't feel well.

32
So is a cat.

33
You can withstand an amazing amount of pain.

34
If you have had lymph nodes removed make sure to do your arm exercises in the hours and days after your surgery. You might feel you can't move but you have to make yourself.

35
Not everyone who gets breast cancer surgery gets swelling in their arm (called lymphedema) no matter what people tell you.

36
You spend more time taking your clothes off and putting them back on than you do getting radiation treatment.

37

If you are going to have chemotherapy, get a warm afghan or stadium blanket to take with you.

38
It's easier to vomit if you've had something to eat. And just because you haven't eaten don't think you won't throw up.

39
If you're tired, lie down. Fighting the urge to rest will only make you irritable.

40
There will be new research and new treatment methods. Don't beat yourself up about what you chose to do. It was your best option at the time.

41
Always keep your insurance cards and ID in your wallet but make sure someone else has copies too.

42
If you get diarrhea, eat bananas, yogurt and applesauce.

43
Drink more water and less alcohol.

44
Buy some really cute pajamas that you can lounge around in all day. If you don't want to spend money on them tell friends who ask what you need that's what you need.

45

You'll start staring at women's breasts. This will pass. Unless you did it before you had cancer.

46

Don't ignore your gut, but don't be ruled by it.

47

Give more weight to science than you do to rumor.

48

Some drugs work well. Sleeping pills, anti-anxiety drugs, antidepressants and pain killers were invented for a reason. If you need them, use them.

49

Call your doctor when you have a question. If he or she doesn't call you back soon, get another doctor.

50

Cry if you want or need to.

51

Don't wear a wig or a hat if you don't want to.

52

A wig does not have to be hot or itch. If it does, something is wrong. See a wig specialist.

53

Make a list of all the medications, vitamins and supplements you take including the dosages. Take that list with you to every appointment.

54

The first time you fill out a new patient form, ask for a copy. Take the copy to every appointment with a new doctor so you can use it to speed up filling out the next one.

55

Enlist a care partner -- husband, spouse or friend -- to help you keep track of appointments and instructions and help you through.

56

Make sure you trust your care partner, share everything about your treatment with her and allow her to talk to your caretakers.

57

Remember, you can get through this, really you can.

58

Make sure you have a comfortable place to rest in your home that's not the bed. A sofa, big comfy chair or a rocker can work.

59
Cancer can get lonely, have a friend go with you to chemotherapy treatments. Play cards. Talk. Or just sit silently and hold hands.

60
Drink lots of water. If you don't like water, try sports drinks or vitamin waters.

61
Sometimes call a friend and start the conversation or by saying, "Let's talk about anything but breast cancer."

Stage III

Recovery

Get over it.

62

Play the cancer card. You don't have to turn it up all the time, just when you think you need it and it will trump anything else on the table.

63

Your hair will grow back. Sometimes better than it was before.

64

Other hair will come back too. Except maybe not your underarm hair.

65

If your health care provider won't accept payment plans, get a new one.

66

Don't second-guess your life. You can't change that you worked in a dry cleaner, ate processed meat, didn't have kids, or took hormones. What's done is done; don't dwell on it.

67

Sleep as much as you need to.

68

Yes everyone IS looking at your breasts. They want to know which one it is – if you had a lumpectomy or a mastectomy. Toy with them. Remember when you were a kid and you knew a secret the other kids didn't? But after a while mention which one it is, or if it's both and what kind of surgery you had. That way they can start making eye contact again.

69

You're the one going through breast cancer, but remember people who love you might be stressed out a little bit too.

70

Take your medicine as prescribed.

71

If your medicine is making you too sick and you can't deal with the symptoms, talk to your doctor about it. If he or she dismisses the complaints, find another doctor.

72

If you share a bed with someone, ask him or her to sleep somewhere else when you are having trouble sleeping.

73

When new studies or drugs or techniques come out that weren't there for you when you had your breast cancer don't feel cheated. Be thankful for the women who won't go through what you went through.

74

After you've had a mastectomy, don't think, "I should have had a lumpectomy."

75

"Chemo brain" is real. It doesn't last. And even if it does, you'll learn to compensate for it.

76

Some people may never acknowledge you have breast cancer. That's their problem, not yours.

77

Remember not to carry heavy things on the side where you had your surgery.

78

If you get nausea, eat crackers and try sucking on crystallized ginger.

79

Try snacking all day instead of eating regular meals. You may have lost your appetite and this will help keep your energy up.

80

If people want to pray for you, say Mass for you or put you in their prayer chain, let them. Even if you're an agnostic or an atheist. If your friends feel better, you will too.

81

If you don't want to talk to someone about your cancer, you don't have to. You don't owe them an explanation.

82

It's not the time to make big changes in your life. Don't quit your job, run off to Europe, get married or start a business. There will be plenty of time for that later. Stress is not your friend right now.

83

Even if you've never been the type to get a massage, it really might make you feel better, so you should try it at least once with someone who specializes in massage for women who have had breast cancer.

84

Every woman looks fabulous in a hat. If you lost your hair and have to wear a hat, you will look fabulous too.

85
You might feel like you are not yourself and you will never be again. But you will.

86
Start exercising. Anything, walking, running, biking, swimming. It doesn't matter what you do but you should do it.

Stage IV

Surviving

Forget about it.

87

If you don't want to call yourself a survivor, don't.
You will survive but it won't change who you are.

88

Bill collectors can be nasty. But you've made it
through cancer. Bill collectors can't compare.

89

If medical bills are overwhelming, see an attorney.

90

Every ache, pain or body change is not the cancer
coming back. You had aches and pains before cancer
and will have them after. Before you blamed them on
too much golf or sleeping in the wrong position.
Those same reasons still work.

91

Some women live for decades with Stage IV cancer.

92

You will improve. That improvement could be
temporary or permanent. Since you don't know
which, believe it will last forever.

93

You didn't want to join the breast cancer club. But
now that you're in, you've got members everywhere
you go. For the rest of your life when you are in a
group of women you'll meet another survivor of
breast cancer.

94

When people ask about your lifestyle in order to figure out why you got cancer they are only looking for order in the universe. Ignore them.

95

There will come a day when someone asks which breast you had cancer in and you'll have to think about it.

96

It's okay if you don't like pink. You don't have to do ribbons and logo-emblazoned T-shirts. If you prefer the item without the breast cancer ribbon, buy it.

97

There will be advances in breast cancer. Don't look back. They weren't there when you had cancer. Be happy for the women coming after you.

98

You'll be inspired by the women who have overcome breast cancer. You'll be surprised by all the women who have had breast cancer and you didn't know. It makes you realize life goes on.

99

Now might be the time to make big changes in your life. Change jobs, run off to Europe, get married or start a business. Do things you've always wanted to do but never had the nerve. You've won, enjoy it.

Acknowledgments

Many thanks are due my friends Francesca Donlan and Dayna Harpster for motivating me to finish this project. If it weren't for their deadlines, this book would have been stuck around number 26.

I want to thank all the people who helped me through cancer. My doctors Lea Blackwell, Alan Brown, Frank Rodriguez and Heather Han were the best and put up with a very obsessive and difficult patient.

I owe a major debt to my friend and golf partner Anne Parnell, who led me to Dara Leichter, who may not have saved my life but certainly saved my sanity.

And with all my heart and soul, I want to thank my husband Rodney Williams who stood by me and helped me through my cancer journey. I could have never made it without him and will be forever grateful for the love he showed me when I was at my least lovable.

About the Author

Melanie Payne is an award-winning journalist and columnist for The News-Press where she writes the consumer column "Tell Mel." She lives in sunny Southwest Florida with her husband Rodney Williams and father Bill Payne.

Other books by Melanie Payne:
Champions Cheaters and Childhood Dreams: Memories of the Soap Box Derby, 2003, University of Akron Press

The Retiree's Guide to Avoiding Scams and Rip-Offs: Advice from Tell Mel (publication: Fall 2012)